How to Start a *Successful* Medical Billing Business

By Alice Scott &
Michele Redmond

Copyright 2022

This publication provides our opinion in regards to starting a medical billing business. We in no way intend to render legal, accounting or any other professional advice.

This publication provides our opinion in regards to starting a medical billing business. We in no way intend to render legal, accounting or any other professional advice.

The authors disclaim any personal liability, loss or risk incurred as a result of using our advice, information, or methods, either directly or indirectly.

Revised January 2022

Copyright 2006 - 2022
8251 New Floyd Rd
Rome, NY 13440
(315)-207-4222
(315)533-4377 fax

Table of Contents

Introduction

The purpose of this book is to help the reader to avoid some of the mistakes we made in starting our medical billing service in 1994. Prior to starting our business, Michele had worked for five years for an insurance company processing medical claims, and I had run my own business for over 25 years.

With our experience we thought it would be no problem, but boy did we have a lot to learn. We purchased an expensive package which was supposed to teach us everything we needed to know to make a fortune at medical billing, but unfortunately the program was a total loss.

This did not stop us. We persisted, we learned much, and finally made our business a success, but we learned the hard way mostly by trial and error. You too can be a success at medical billing by learning from our experiences and avoiding our mistakes.

In today's economy many people are looking for work, especially work that they can do from home. Some are just looking for a part time job and some want to start a business that will serve them for years. This book will help to know if a medical billing service is the right business for you.

You will need to learn what equipment is needed to start your service, how to choose software, how to find clients, what to charge, what to say and do on your first appointment, what your work actually consists of, what you need to know about codes, and how to actually get started as a medical biller.

We talk to many people who want to start a medical billing business and they want to know if it is possible to accomplish. It is definitely possible – we are proof of that and we've met many others who started the same as we did and are now running their own business.

But it is important to know what it will take so that you can properly prepare. Many of those people that we talk to tell me that they want to start a medical billing business so they are taking a class now on medical coding. My question to them is do you want to start a medical billing business or a medical coding business? Medical billing and coding are so closely associated when you do a search on the internet that people just assume that medical coding must be learned to do medical billing. While it can be an asset to a billing service to have a certified coder on staff, it is not necessary. Taking a coding class first is not the right way to get started.

There are so many other things that are more important to look at before thinking about things like medical coding. More important to consider is how much money will you need to invest to get started, how long will it be before you can write a paycheck to yourself, where will your business be located, how will you choose the right equipment and software, and do you have some background in medical billing?

What is a day in the life of the owner of a medical billing service like? First of all, this is not a data entry job although there is a lot of data entry. You also have to be a bit of a detective to deal with all the issues that come up every day. It also depends at what stage you are at in your business. When first starting out all your time should be spent finding clients.

Many beginners want to spend their time shopping for furniture and setting up their office. You definitely want to have work space laid out efficiently but without clients you don't have a business so we say start looking. Finding clients is the most difficult part of this business for most beginners so you need to get out there and find some to get started. Lack of clients is also the main reason most business fail.

We are often asked how long it takes to find the first clients and for many it is several months. It doesn't surprise me when someone tells me they have been looking for clients for six months and don't have one yet. Many people think the doctors will come knocking on their door looking for them but this is not how it works. In the beginning you can expect to spend several hours a day working on marketing.

Once you are up and running a typical day may involve picking up work from your local providers. We do this once a week. We try to get any claims out the same day as they come in so we are entering new patients and their claims first. Once we get the claims entered, we batch the ones that can go electronically and send them to the clearinghouse. We print out any remaining ones that go on paper. Many clearinghouses will submit any necessary claims on paper also.

When the claims are done, we download any ERAs or Electronic Remittance Advice. These are payments for the claims that were sent electronically. We then enter payments from the EOBs the provider sent us. This is where a lot of the detective work comes in. Often insurance claims are denied for a variety of reasons and we generally spend the rest of the day figuring out these issues and dealing with them. If there is any extra time it is spent running aging reports and calling or checking websites to see why these claims are not processed yet.

Once a month we run the patient billing. This involves sending statements to any of the patients who have outstanding balances. Sometimes we are signing up a provider for permission to use the different insurance carrier's websites. Once a week we mail out all our paper insurance claims. The duties are varied and there is always a lot to do.

We made a lot of mistakes in starting our business. There was no information available for us to learn from. Although many of our mistakes are embarrassing, we will share them so you don't make the same ones we did. We want to shorten your learning curve by showing you what worked for us and what didn't.

This book is designed to give all the information you will need to get off to a great start. It will **not** teach you how to do medical billing, but it **will** teach you to start a *successful* medical billing business. Best of luck in your new venture!!

Our Story

Michele and I started our medical billing service in 1994. When I first saw an ad for medical billing at home, I gave it to my daughter, Michele, who had been working for a major health insurance company for the last 5 years at a very stressful job. She called the number and received an informational packet about a medical billing package that cost around $5000.

She was ready to start a family and wanted to work at home, but she had never run her own business. That's where I came in. I had run my own business for over 25 years and was now looking for a new opportunity. I didn't know anything about insurance billing, but we figured as a team, we would be great.

We sent away for several other packets on similar packages and we started comparing the offers and found they ranged in price from $4000 to $10,000 and in training from two days to five days.

Some companies offered their own clearinghouses which seemed like a savings although we were not sure what a clearinghouse was. Most offered the necessary software. We spent a lot of time comparing companies, checking with the Better Business Bureau, and doing research to see what would be our best option.

We chose a company in Atlanta that charged $5000 and booked our flights for the two-day training. We were excited. However, after the two-day training, we didn't know much more about this business than before we went.

The package was useless. The software was produced by the company itself; therefore, it was not compatible with any clearinghouse other than their own, which wasn't sending any claims electronically at that time. They were sending the claims on paper.

We didn't get any useful information from them as far as starting our business, actually doing medical billing, getting accounts or doing follow up. Most of the time was spent training us on their software.

Now we were $10,000 in debt and still at square one. We started over. After logging on to a bulletin board service strictly for medical billing, we received a lot of information on different software and clearinghouses. We sent for demos and purchased Lytec Medical and Dental software.

We got some marketing tips and made a few friends. We did anything and everything we could think of to get some clients. When we say anything and everything, we mean it. We were very creative in our initial marketing.

Our first account was a new doctor who knew less about insurance billing than we did, which turned out to be a blessing. We didn't make much money, but we were getting experience and that's what we needed.

Medical billing was much different at that time than it is today. The internet was new and did not have a lot of information available on the subject. Packages such as the one we purchased were very common and mostly scams that preyed on people like us who just wanted to start their own business.

We made some mistakes in the beginning because we had nowhere to find information. We learned a lot by trial and error, and we had a few laughs along the way. Now people call us all the time asking for our advice on getting started in their own medical billing business.

We decided the best way to share the information was to put it all together in a manual - exactly "how to" start and run a *successful* medical billing business. We wrote this manual so you can refer to it often when your next question comes up.

It contains what is actually needed to get started and build a successful business. With our success we found a desire to help others get off to a great start.

We have revised this book quite a few times to keep up with the changes in the industry. What worked a few years ago is antiquated now and there is a need to put new systems into place.

Technology has changed a lot in the last few years offering the medical biller many new ways to save time and money. Changes are constant in this industry and it is important that information is up to date. This business is constantly changing and with the change is the necessity to keep up and stay competitive. It is important that the beginner know what he or she is getting into and what to expect in this business.

Getting Started

The key to any successful business is research. In order to establish a successful business, a good foundation must be built. Without a good solid foundation, the business will crumble to the ground with the first challenge it faces. In order to build a good foundation, you must research the field of medical billing thoroughly. It is crucial to completely understand the business if you are going to succeed.

There are several places to go to begin your research. One of the best places to get information on medical billing services is from other people who have already done it.

This book is a great place to start! It is one of the main reasons we wrote it. When we started, we tried to talk to other local services. We didn't look at it as being competitive. Unfortunately, they did! This is a very competitive business but there are some in this field willing to help others. We have met other billing service owners at a local insurance seminar who were located about 1 ½ hours away from us and they were open to sharing information. If you can find a way to connect with someone in person, whether local or a little way away, it could be very helpful.

Another place to find other medical billers who will share information is on the internet. Watch the medical billing forums for great questions and answers to the problems we are dealing with every day. Our very active forum is located at www.medicalbillinglive.com/forum. We get some great threads going on marketing, starting your business, and getting your first clients. Our readers are not afraid to share their experiences and knowledge.

Websites for software can be accessed and actually download demos to find one that you are comfortable with. You can shop for office furniture and supplies. You can research medical billing courses and even take courses online.

This business can give the freedom you may be looking for. You set your own hours so you can start your business while you are still working. We've seen many people start their business by finding a client and doing the work at night after they get home from work. We've also seen a lady who worked for a medical billing service decide that she wanted to start her own business and she had it up and running within months of her decision.

Many medical billers work from home and raise their children around their work. Some are just looking for a little extra money to help out with the family finances and many are single mothers who must provide for their families. It is a very flexible business.

The most difficult part of this business for most beginners is signing up those first clients. It's not the work involved or learning the new software. It's signing up providers. If you are determined to make this business work for you, nothing will stop you and you will learn how to find the new clients. Much of the success of this business depends on the willingness of the individual to persevere. He or she must overcome all the obstacles that will appear.

Today there are many places to find help with questions in the medical billing field. There are many courses available, including ours, books to read, and websites to gather information. Choices are better than ever in software and equipment.

See what it takes to get your business up and running. Besides our free forum, we offer a subscription to our free newsletter offering information on current topics at http://www.solutions-medical-billing.com. We will help you get started. You can also find more of our ebooks available at www.medicalbillinglive.com.

Billing Knowledge

Billing knowledge is critical to success in this business. You must have some background or be willing to learn by taking a good medical billing course. Much of the work of doing medical billing is fixing problems and facing new issues. Without knowledge of how the process works it is easy to get lost.

There are many places to get an education on medical insurance billing. This is indispensable in this business. One of the best options is to take a course in medical billing. If you decide to take a course, make sure it is taught by someone who has actually done medical billing. Check out what the courses actually offer as many are very expensive and offer much information that is never used by a biller.

This fact made us realize the need for a practical medical billing course designed to give the student the necessary knowledge to obtain a job as a biller in a medical office, a clinic or a hospital or to start their own business. In 2013 we started designing just such a certified course and now offer it at www.medicalbillingstudycourse.com, There are 10 certified courses that can be purchased individually or in a package.

In running our medical billing business for the last 20 years we have hired several employees after they graduated from a medical billing school or course. Never have we found a person prepared for the work that they will face. We had to continue training these employees for as long as a year after their courses for them to understand what is required to do a good job. One lady we hired had spent two years and over $9000.00 to get her degree but she was a beginner with very limited knowledge as far as we were concerned.

We realized that most medical billing courses are developed by teachers and people not actually working in a billing office and their knowledge of billing is nowhere near the requirements of the job. We took the years of training employees experience and designed an eight-course online training to give the student just the info they will need to succeed along with two additional courses on starting and marketing a medical billing business.

Michele got most of her education by working for the insurance company and I got mine by listening to her. Whatever you choose, make sure you understand medical billing inside and out.

Good experience can be obtained working in a doctor's office doing the billing. Even if it is billing for a medical specialty practice, it will be extremely beneficial. Nothing beats actual experience.

A good understanding of medical billing is necessary. Also, the ability to read an explanation of benefits to know if it was paid correctly and how to act on it if it is not paid correctly. Much of this comes with experience.

Computer and Printer

The computer or computers are our livelihood. Computers get outdated very quickly, so don't buy the one that just meets your requirements. Do not use the business computer for a personal computer as well. The information on your computer must be protected and using it for personal needs will compromise the safety.

Be prepared to upgrade the computer system at least every four years. Make sure it has a good backup system as it is very important to keep the information backed up daily.

Make sure to consider all that will be needed in a computer. Besides size of the hard drive and memory you will need a high-speed connection, a good virus protection, a firewall and a modem. If you expect to be more than a one-person business it will require more than one computer with networking between them. A good IT person to deal with problems that arise is also necessary.

A decent size monitor is a must. Remember, many hours will be spent looking at that screen. Many billers have more than one monitor hooked up to their computer to be able to view more than one screen at a time. We furnish at least two monitors for our workers and a few have three.

The printer is also very important as a lot of printing is required. You may have thought you wouldn't need a printer as everything goes electronic, but that is not reality. Many secondary claims must be printed. Most no fault and workers comp claims must be printed. EOBs must be photocopied and submitted with secondary and tertiary claims.

Make sure the printer meets all of the printing needs and is economical to operate. It can be difficult to calculate the cost of printing as many printers don't advertise that information, but the information is usually available on the internet and is important. You will find yourself making many photocopies and want them to be made at a reasonable cost.

Know what type of forms that will be printed. A laser printer is a little more expensive to buy, but saves you a lot in cartridges. When we first started, we had to print 3-part Workers Comp forms so we had to use a dot matrix printer. Fortunately, these forms are no longer required so we switched to a much more efficient laser printer.

This printer had two drawers plus a feed tray. It was very convenient as we keep CMS 1500 forms in one drawer and plain paper in another. But then that printer became outdated. We next used a large 4 drawer printer/scanner/copier that we rented that did things we never thought of and at a cost of only 1.4 cents per copy. Machines like this can be rented fairly reasonably. We now use Brother printers with two drawers.

We used to offer credentialing services to providers. This is where we found some great advantages to the new printer. We could now scan a credentialing packet after it was completed and email or fax it to a provider right from the printer. As printers progressed, we find we can now do all of that on our Brother printers.

Now we have the ability to scan any document and email or fax it wherever we please. This opened up a huge number of possibilities to us. It is amazing the uses we find for this machine. The ability to scan documents allows us to scan claims and EOBs and store them on the computer rather than in file cabinets.

If you need to print your own business cards or brochures to get started, you may need a color printer. Many of us who love photography have digital cameras with a color printer for the photos. You can use this printer to make business cards and brochures. Carefully think about what you will be printing when making your decisions.

Practice Management System

There are many good software programs available for medical billing. The big difference between practice management systems today is whether they are server based or web-based. Server based software is installed on your computer while web-based software is accessed on the internet.

The biggest advantage of a web-based practice management system is that it can be accessed from anywhere. You don't have to be on the computer in your office. This allows both the provider and the biller to access the same program. The provider's office can look up a patient's balance without calling the biller to find out what it is. Your provider can run reports on the software system you are using.

The software package (practice management system) can cost several thousand dollars and if server based it must be updated every two or three years. Changes in the industry make it necessary to update to accommodate these changes. An example is the change from ICD9 to ICD10 codes in 2014. The change to ICD10s involved the change from four diagnosis codes on a claim to as many as twelve. The software must be updated in order to accommodate this. So, if the software is not updated the claims would not be able to be sent any longer once the ICD10s were implemented.

We have used NDC Lytec Medical for many years which is server based. They are reasonably priced and easy to use and kept up with our needs. There are many advantages to a web-based program but they can be expensive. In recent years many new web-based programs have come out that are more reasonable so it is important to do lots of research prior to deciding on software. Lytec does now offer a web-based software as well as the server based.

Make sure to start out with a practice management system that you are happy with as it is a huge deal to change systems. This is one of the main reasons we have not changed to a web-based program. All the information in the old system will have to be transferred to the new system and there are generally a lot of glitches when a transfer like this is attempted.

Demo's of practice management systems can often be downloaded from the Internet. Make sure you choose a software program that you are comfortable using and meets your requirements. You will most likely want it to handle more than one provider's work. Also available are some specialty software programs for chiropractic, mental health, physical therapy, etc. Remember that these programs are limited to those specialties.

Some of our providers require that we work on their web-based programs. So many of our accounts are in our Lytec system and a few we connect to. We can generally learn a new system pretty quickly. We have even talked to billers who don't have their own systems but only use the providers systems. This is unusual as some providers do not even have a practice management system.

In software terms, do you need a single user or multi-user software? Multi-user software can be accessed by more than one person at a time. For example, Lytec is available for one user, up to five users, or up to 10 users. You don't want to buy a single-user software if you plan for your business to grow and have more than one user. Or at least make sure you can upgrade to the multi-user version without too much hassle or cost.

There are many things to take into consideration when choosing the software. Do you plan on doing all the billing yourself or do you want to grow into a larger billing service with multiple employees? It is a big deal to have to change software in the future and try to get all the information transferred from one program to another.

Web-based software is available with price based upon how much volume is expected. Your agreement with the software vendor will probably lock you into a certain time frame, probably a commitment to a year's service.

There are many different ways of pricing web-based software so make sure to be clear on total costs including clearinghouse charges. Some web-based software is priced per seat or by how many computers will be accessing it at the same time. Some are priced by the number of providers you have.

When comparing software check to see if they come with CPT and ICD10 codes available to import. This isn't a big deal when billing for small specialty providers, but if when billing for a larger medical practice – this can be huge. Entering all the ICD10 or ICD10 (diagnosis) codes and CPT (procedure) codes can be tedious. Lytec now offers a service called Encoder Pro that will look up codes to make sure they are valid. This is a very nice feature we use often.

Software is not something purchased and that's it. If you are in business for any amount of time (hopefully you aren't doing this for a six-month time filler!!) you will need to update your software if it is server based. Web-based software is being updated all the time.

The world of medical billing is constantly changing especially since HIPAA. The practice management system must be able to change with it. That's one of the great things about web-based software. It can be changed on an ongoing basis not just when a new version is released.

Another important reason to pick a good solid company to purchase your software from is for support. You may find yourself in a position where you can't get your software to do something you need it to, or you are having a problem with your software. You will need to be able to contact the company for support and the support needs to be good.

When you purchase your software, find out if you are purchasing it directly from the company or from a reseller. Usually the price is the same, but the reseller may offer support that the company doesn't.

When a medical billing package is purchased that comes with software, check to see if that software is compatible to any clearinghouse or if you will be locked into using their clearinghouse which may not fit your needs. See our chapter on Clearinghouses. Choose the software and clearinghouses carefully. They are big decisions to make.

Once you have your software installed in your computer, or have accessed your web-based program, practice with it. Learn to get around in your program. Enter some fictitious claims. See how the program works. Read the manual from cover to cover. Familiarize yourself completely with the program. You need to get comfortable with using the software.

In our original search for web-based software, we found most were cost prohibitive for our needs. We were billing for about 60 providers at that time and many companies charged a monthly fee per doctor that was more than we charged some of our smaller providers. We would have had to give up all our small accounts in order to make it work. On top of that most of these companies charged a hefty upfront fee ranging from $5000 to $22,000. It was out of the question. But today with more competition you may find a good one at a reasonable cost.

Other software you may require are a word processing program such as Word or Microsoft Office. We often use Publisher and Excel spreadsheets for different projects. We also use QuickBooks to keep our financial records and to bill our providers.

Clearinghouses

In order to submit claims electronically, a method must be chosen to transmit the claims to the insurance companies. There are a couple of different options available. One of these options is using the services of a clearinghouse. The other is using free software offered by the individual insurance carriers.

Clearinghouses have changed a lot in the past few years. They now offer many more services with bigger benefits for the user. Costs vary greatly between different clearinghouses, so calculate the estimates carefully when making a decision.

Many times, a practice management system will be tied to a particular clearinghouse. This doesn't necessarily mean that particular software **must** use that clearinghouse but it is important to find out. They may strongly encourage the use of the clearinghouse they are linked to but it may be possible to submit to other clearinghouses if you choose.

When claims are sent through a clearinghouse, they are routed electronically to the appropriate insurance company. The clearinghouse acts as a middleman. Most clearinghouses post the list of payers or insurance companies that they submit to on their website.

Many clearinghouses offer services in addition to just electronic claims submission. Some offer online eligibility, electronic remittances, and claim status checking. It is important that you know all the services you will be signing up for and the fees you will be charged.

Sometimes the print to paper is an option offered for an additional cost by the clearinghouse. Any paper claims that cannot go electronically are then printed and stuffed into envelopes and mailed directly to the insurance carrier by the clearinghouse.

Some insurance companies offer free software that will allow you to submit claims to them electronically. Usually, the free software option means double entry of the data. It is usually a standalone program and you have to enter all of the data in your practice management program for tracking purposes and in the stand-alone program to submit the claims.

Other insurance carriers have an online claim submission option through their website. Once a person is registered claims can be directly submitted through the website. This is also considered electronic submission but will require that the information also be entered in the practice management system for tracking purposes again causing double entry.

A few small insurance companies do not have the capability to receive insurance claims electronically. These companies generally require that their claims be submitted on CMS 1500 forms.

The clearinghouse will do this for you for a charge, it's called turning them to paper, but it may be more efficient and cheaper to print those on paper (CMS 1500 forms) and send them directly to the insurance company yourself. Compare the clearinghouse fee to your expenses. When printing and mailing yourself, you can fit many claims in one envelope if they are all going to the same address.

Decide the most practical method of sending the claims electronically and be willing to change if a better method becomes available. One thing you will learn about this business is that things are always changing and it is important that you stay aware of the changes and keep up with technology.

In choosing a clearinghouse there are several things you will be looking for.

✓ Do they have a minimum requirement?

✓ Is there a set-up fee?

✓ What is the cost per claim?

✓ What do they charge to turn a claim to paper?

✓ Do you get confirmation that the claims went?

✓ Do they submit to the carriers that your providers bill?

✓ What type of error reports do they send you?

✓ What type of scrubber do they have for up front editing to prevent claims from being denied?

✓ How will the clearinghouse bill you?

✓ If you have a problem and need to speak to someone, how do they answer phone calls or do you have to leave a message?

CMS 1500, UB04 and Workers Comp forms

Even when sending claims electronically, CMS 1500 forms are still needed. They are the standard red and white insurance claim filing form used by most medical providers and insurance carriers. CMS 1500 forms can vary greatly in price and are less expensive when purchased in larger quantities.

Workers comp insurance claims must be filed differently. In NY they are not filed on CMS 1500 forms but a special form called a C4 which is available from the Workers Comp Dept. website. Whenever filing a workers comp insurance claim, this C4 form must be completed. Rules for filing workers comp claims vary from state to state.

In NY there are currently two separate C4 forms available. One is for the initial visit and reports how the accident occurred and what is involved. The second form is for subsequent visits. Physical therapists and occupational therapists file workers' comp claims on a slightly different single page form called an OT/PT-4.

Once a workers comp claim form is completed, we print two copies. We send one to the insurance company and the other goes to the workers comp office. We do not keep copies of these forms since we can print another one easier than to find one in a file cabinet if we need to resubmit.

Some software actually creates the C4 form and you only need to print them on white paper. If your software does not print the form, you can usually download a form off the internet and print your own.

The forms may also be purchased preprinted. Check with the State Workers Comp Board to find where to order these forms.

UB04 forms are used for hospital and facility billing. Facilities include drug and alcohol rehab centers, eating disorder clinics, hospitals and ambulatory surgery centers. Not all practice management systems are capable of printing UB04 forms. When doing facility billing on UB04 forms make sure the practice management system has that capability.

Internet

The internet can be a very useful tool in starting your medical billing business. As stated in the previous section, much research can be done on the internet. In doing that research, you may make some contacts that you will want to stay in touch with as you establish your business.

Most insurance companies have websites that the biller, as the provider's representative, will need to access. Some of these websites offer a convenient place to check benefits on patients, verify ID#s, check claims status, submit adjustment forms, and much more. Many companies have their newsletters and/or bulletins available on-line. The newsletters contain valuable information regarding billing and should be read.

Many forms are available on these websites that are useful. When a provider wants to become participating with the insurance company or needs to update or change information, the forms are usually available on-line.

Most clearinghouses use the internet to receive claim files. The claims are batched into a file by the practice management system and uploaded to the clearinghouse via the internet.

We also use the internet to look up NPI numbers, phone numbers of an insurance company or a doctor if we do not have it on file. We've also found it very handy when we need to send flowers or a gift to a provider.

As you can see, the internet is an important tool in starting a medical billing business. Also important is having a high-speed connection. Of course, having the internet connection opens up your medical billing data to viruses and hackers. Make sure to have good virus protection, pop-up blockers, firewalls, spam blockers, malware, etc. to ensure proper security for your information.

Phones and phone lines

You will find you require at least two phone lines - one land line or cell phone for your telephone and another for your computer and fax machine. High speed internet is a must for your internet needs.

We prefer a land line rather than a cell phone for our business needs. Cell calls can be very staticky, noisy and unreliable. When a potential client is on the phone you want to be sure to have a clear connection. Besides if you have employees you will want to be able to have them have phone access and also be able to transfer calls, etc.

Keep a personal phone line separate from your business line. You do not want to have your business line tied up with personal calls. Do not allow children to answer your business phone unless you have trained them to do it in a professional manner and they are capable of taking a message and getting it fully in tact to you.

Check the various services available with your phone company. Before we went to the digital phone service, we have now we had rollover on our first line which means that if we are talking on line one, another incoming call will automatically rollover to the second line if it is not in use.

You will find that physician's offices do not like to call and get a busy signal so you want to make sure you have at least two lines available. Once we started hiring employees, we eventually found it necessary to add a third and fourth and fifth phone line which we then used for the computer modems and outgoing calls so our other lines were not tied up.

Get yourself at least one good two (or more) line phone. There are many options available and phones are relatively inexpensive now. We also find that a headset is invaluable for getting work done while you are on hold with an insurance company. A speakerphone option is also a must for us.

As you grow, you may want to consider a phone system. The initial cost is a little high, but if you grow to have several employees and you're not all sitting in one big room, a phone system is great. It allows you to intercom between phones, transfer calls, and have individual voice mails. Before we switched over, we would have to yell to each other when a phone call came in! It was not very professional.

We were lucky with our first phone system. We bought it used from a provider we billed for who had shut down an office. If you find yourself ready for a phone system and cost is an issue, watch the classifieds for a used one or even check eBay and Craig's List.

A few years ago, we changed our whole phone system once again. It is important to keep up with the changes in technology to find the best alternative to your needs. Our phone bill was getting very expensive so we started looking into the options.

Our local charges for the five phone lines was over $250 per month. Our long-distance charges including our 1-800 line had grown to over $200 per month. We were spending almost $500 per month for our phones.

Our office manager looked into the options and decided on a voice over computer system where there were no long-distance charges. All calls were included in the monthly fee along with voice mail for each phone. There was also no need for all the extra lines. Each phone will be accessible at the same time without the use of extra lines.

The exciting part about this new system besides the savings is that we won't have to answer the phone any more unless the call is directed to our individual extension. Sometimes our phones were ringing all day. These constant interruptions to the girls answering the calls and transferring them to the correct person were interfering with productivity.

There are times that you will be unable to answer the phone. It is very important that the caller is able to leave a message. Set up your voice mail leaving a clear message on your machine with the name of your company and an assurance that their call will be returned in a reasonable time frame. Make sure your message sounds professional

Code Books

Depending on whether your practice management system comes with some type of coder for CPT (or procedure codes) you may need to keep current CPT code books. They are published yearly. Code books cost between $50 and $150. There are many suppliers of these code books. www.amazon.com is a good place to search. CPT codes are copyright protected by the AMA and cannot be copied.

ICD10 codes however are not copyright protected and can be found on various websites by doing a google search for current ICD10 codes. You can also find sites that transfer ICD9 codes to ICD10 codes.

Codes are changing every year and it is necessary to keep on top of them. Depending on the specialties of the providers you work with will determine if you need to order new ones each year.

When only working with some specialties such as chiropractors, you may not need to purchase a CPT book every year.

HCPCS code books may also be required for some providers. HCPCS are another form of CPT codes used for certain services such as drug administration, immunizations, enteral therapy, and durable medical equipment.

Desk, chair, photocopier, and filing cabinet

A good-sized computer desk and comfortable chair are required. You will be spending a lot of time in this chair and want to avoid unnecessary trips to the chiropractor. The desk needs to be large so you can spread out your work.

Also needed is at least one large filing cabinet and lots of file folders to set up a filing system. Much work can now be stored digitally but we find it necessary to keep information on our providers handy.

Claim information will need to be stored that was sent to your office from the provider's office will need to be stored, as well as EOBs and ERAs after they are entered. Later on you may refer occasionally to these files to find certain EOBs to resubmit a secondary claim. Much of this information can be stored digitally.

Legally you must keep this information for a certain length of time, generally three years. If a provider is audited, the biller may be asked for information. When storing everything on paper, it can quickly turn into a large amount of material.

Keep each providers information separate. We keep one folder for claim information, one folder for EOBs, and one folder for the provider information.

When we filed our work in file cabinets, every month we rotate the claims and EOB files so they were current and anything we needed to find from the past could be located. We wrote the dates in large black numbers on the front of each file folder. We would store records for the previous year in file boxes labeled so we could find something if need be.

Now we store everything we can digitally by scanning it, still identifying all materials and dates in folders that can be easily found. We find this works much better than storing all that paper.

A photocopier/scanner/printer will be required for printing claims, making photocopies, faxing and scanning work. Purchase a good one as it hopefully will be doing a lot of work.

Business cards and brochures

Required are some professional looking business cards and brochures. Business cards are relatively inexpensive. You may want to hire a printing and graphics business to do these or you can do them up yourself on your computer very inexpensively.

The benefit to doing them yourself is that you can change them as you need to. You may decide to do a brochure on dental insurance billing to leave at dental offices. A month later you may decide to target physical therapists. This way you are not paying a printer every time you want a small or large change in your brochure.

There are several good publishing programs available to make brochures, fliers, business cards, etc. Check them out in your software store. Microsoft Publisher is one.

There are also some very fancy papers available to dress up your brochure. You can find paper in office supply stores or order by mail from Paper Direct.

When we first started out, we used brochures for a lot of things. We sent them in mailings, we placed them in our local hospital's waiting room, and we handed them out when we made cold calls.

Mailing, Postage & Envelopes

You will find when you mail out your paper insurance claims that you often have several going to the same company. These can be mailed in one envelope as long as they are all going to the same address.

Some companies have several different locations. Make sure you mail to the proper location. Failure to do so can hold up payment on a claim.

When there are four or five claims in an envelope, it is necessary to know the correct amount of required postage. An electronic postage scale will come in very handy. Otherwise, it requires going to the post office, waiting in line, and expecting the postal worker to weigh each envelope for you.

It is really an unnecessary expense to rent a postage meter machine. If you keep first class stamps on hand, you save yourself hundreds of dollars of expense per year in renting a postage meter when the scale is all you really need.

A scale can be purchased very inexpensively one at any office supply store. We usually purchase about a month's worth of stamps at a time. Be sure to purchase stamps to cover extra weight. Our mail varies in weight from less than one ounce to over one pound. We purchase all the necessary stamps to cover these amounts.

Postage rates and requirements change often. It is necessary to keep up with these changes to prevent envelopes from being returned for not enough postage.

Window envelopes designed for CMS 1500's are available in two sizes, one that will hold a few claims and a larger size for a larger batch of claims. We use both. You just fold the CMS forms to fit the envelope with the insurance company address in the window. This saves printing labels.

Even though the majority of our claims are going electronically, we still mail hundreds of claims a week to insurance companies that do not yet accept electronic billing or secondary claims that cannot go electronically.

The best way that we have found to sort these paper claims is a box that we found at an office supply store. It is a cardboard box divided into 21 slots that are just the right size for 8 ½" x 11" claim forms.

We've labeled each slot and as we take the claims out of the printer, we file them into the proper slot. Twice a week we go through the claims, put them in their envelopes and send them off using the scale in our office to apply the proper postage. We can put the claims in our mail box and avoid a trip to the post office.

Legal Issues

Some states (like NJ) require a medical billing service to be registered with the state. In NJ you must complete a registration form and have it approved prior to opening the business. Check to see if there are any requirements in your state.

Make sure to check with local government offices also such as the county clerk to see if there are any restrictions or rules you need to know about. Zoning is another issue to look into. If you want to work from home make sure you are not breaking any zoning laws. If you wish to put up a sign advertising your service there may be restrictions on the size and location of the sign.

You will be required to file tax returns on your business. We suggest you use an accountant unless you are well versed in this area. Tax returns will be filed with a tax identification number which can be either your social security number or an EIN. You can obtain an EIN free of charge online at https://irs-ein-number.com/.

You will need to decide whether you will establish your business as a sole proprietor, corporation or as a partnership. Your accountant and attorney can give you a better idea of how to set up your business. Incorporating as you grow can be a tax advantage your accountant can better explain. It also helps to protect your personal assets.

E&O insurance (errors and omissions) protects you from financial liability from lawsuits from your potential clients and should be considered when starting your business.

Office

One of the first decisions to make will be where to run your business. Will you work out of your home or rent an office?

Most people who start medical billing businesses do so in order to stay at home. When choosing to work at home, an office or space where you can spread out will be required.

If your children will be near when you are working, you will need space for them to be playing quietly while you are on the phone. Don't try to run your business off your kitchen table. With medical billing, it just won't work.

When the decision is made to rent an office, there will be extra expenses from the beginning. Some people feel that it looks more professional to have an outside office. Our feeling is that if you are doing a good job, the doctor doesn't care where you are working.

Wherever you decide to have your office you will need to consider how much space you will need. We have found that we needed several different work stations.

One section to actual work on the computer, another section for filing, and a third section for sending the mail. You will mail any non-electronic claims, secondary claims, patient notes, patient bills, appeals, workers compensation claims, letters and no fault claims. Make sure to take all of this into consideration when choosing a location.

There are many tax advantages in owning your own business. You will need to check with your accountant to make sure you keep track of all the expenses that will be deductible on your income taxes.

Naming your business

The name of the business can be very important. Remember, you will be answering the phone many times a day with this name. Write down all of your choices and then say them out loud. This may seem childish, but it will help you pick a good name.

The name should be relevant to what you are doing, yet it should set you apart from your competition. For example, if you were starting a vending machine business, you wouldn't want to name it Johnson Inc. No one can tell what kind of business it is.

You also wouldn't want to call it Best Vending Machines because that doesn't set you apart from the competition. A name more like Sammy's Snacks would be good. It relates to what you do, but it's personable and different from the competition.

Check out the competition in your area and make sure you don't use an existing name. Check with your county clerk regarding registering your name.

It is also better to not limit yourself by calling your business Johnson's Medical Billing – like we did. You will actually be so much more than a billing service. You will end up consulting and running a full practice management business. Make sure you check with your local county clerk to make sure someone else isn't already using the name you chose.

Clients

The final requirement needed to get your medical billing business started is clients. This can be the most difficult part of the process and one of the most important. There are many different ways to look for clients and we suggest you use several.

You first need to understand that you are asking a provider to trust you with their income. The payments from their insurance claims are very important to them and they do not easily give the job of collecting them to someone they do not know.

Usually, the money does not actually come to you, it still goes directly to the provider, but you are now responsible for making sure that it is paid on time. Situations in each office will differ.

Many times, it is difficult for a provider to let the billing go outside of the office because they feel they are losing control. As more experience is gained, you will see the needs of the office and learn to help the provider overcome the fears they have of hiring a service.

Some providers will already be signed up with a service they but they are not happy. This provider may be looking for someone who can do a better job than what they are now getting. Consider the problems they are experiencing now and convince the doctor why this won't happen if you are doing the billing.

Keep in mind when looking for clients that some offices are so well run that they may not need your services. If one person has been responsible for the billing for a long period of time and has been doing it well, it is very unlikely they will think that you will do a better job.

It's a good idea to introduce yourself and let them know what you do, as eventually the situation in the office may change and they may be looking for an alternative. Also, you never know where a referral may come from.

Sometimes at first glance an office will appear to be running well, but upon a closer look you will find they have serious problems. In most of these cases, they don't want to admit that they have any problems. If you clearly see some issues, try to approach them from that angle but do it tactfully. They may be sensitive to the issue.

See our section on marketing to learn how to get clients.

Understanding Your Value to Providers

It is important to understand what it is that you do that makes you valuable to a provider's office. Until you really understand this, it is difficult to convince a provider that they should hire you. Providers can hire help to send claims directly from their own office. Why should they hire you?

Very few offices are still sending claims on paper but there are a few. One of these might hire you simply because they want their claims to go electronically so they are getting paid quicker. They've found it complicated to do this from their office or maybe they don't even have a computer. In some cases, they've tried to do it electronically from the office and it didn't work out well.

You must know the requirements of each insurance company, make sure all data on the claim is correct, including the coding and follow up on any unpaid or rejected claims. A billing professional knows how to get claims paid quickly and correctly and knows how to make sure a provider is getting paid the most for his or her services.

You may get a provider to sign with you because he or she can't keep good knowledgeable help in their office. A new provider just out of school trying to open their own practice may hire you because he is keeping down costs of additional help at the beginning.

The longer you work in this profession, the better you will understand how valuable you can be to your providers. You will eventually consider yourself a consultant. As you gain experience in your field of billing, you will be able to offer suggestions to increase their income (and yours) and improve their efficiency.

An office may contact you because their receivables are way too low and they can't seem to figure out how to increase them. We once met with a doctor who owned a family practice with three MDs and three NPs. They were a very busy office seeing 80-100 patients a day but they were barely bringing in enough to keep the doors open.

The doctor himself wasn't even getting paid. Yet we had to convince him he needed us. Within six months of hiring us we increased his receivables 100%. As you can imagine, we are now invaluable to him. Anyone can send claims to an insurance company, but it takes a professional to do medical billing. There is so much more to billing than just submitting the claims.

You are not just a billing service; you are a billing professional and also a consultant. You will not just submit claims for your providers, but you will maximize their receivables. You will make sure they get reimbursed for their services.

Assure them that you do not loose claims to timely filing and that you follow through on all claims to get them paid. Remember, depending on how you are charging your providers, your income can be directly dependent to how much money you collect for the provider.

There are many ways to become invaluable to the providers in addition to doing a great job on their billing. You can act as a consultant to them advising them of ways they can increase their receivables such as making sure they are billing more than the allowed amount of the insurance companies. Providers also are looking for help with credentialing or recredentialing and address changes.

Many providers cringe at the sight of paperwork and they are very grateful to you for helping them out. Any of these little things that can be done to help them out just helps to build a stronger loyalty which usually leads to a long-term relationship.

One of our best accounts is an office with two doctors who had placed an ad in the local paper for a person with billing experience. We answered the ad and after talking to the doctor, he realized that if he hired us it would eliminate the need for a workspace for a new employee, a computer, and all the additional expenses of another employee.

We've been working with them for over 20 years now and they are thrilled and give great referrals for us. They don't hesitate to tell others how much money they save and how much we have increased their income.

Marketing

Marketing is the most important part of getting a billing business started. Without clients, there is no business. There are many ways to market a new business, but the most important thing is to keep an open mind to all possibilities. There is no one right way to market.

If you're new to this, it is a good idea to try many different techniques and find what you are comfortable with and what works for you. Whatever methods are used, it is best to be direct and honest.

We are always finding new ways to market. Referrals are by far the best, but when you don't have any clients yet, it is hard to find anyone to refer you.

The absolutely best way to market is by networking. You need to get out and meet people – people in the medical field. It is much easier to talk to someone about what you do at a social event than trying to get past a gatekeeper to talk to the boss.

Look through our chapter on marketing and keep your mind open. You may think of any idea we haven't tried yet. For more ideas and techniques on marketing check out our two ebooks on marketing "Twelve Marketing Strategies to Grow Your Medical Billing Business" and "Advanced Medical Billing Marketing for the New Economy"

1. ***Start with the doctors you go to***. Ask your family practitioner how he is currently doing his billing? Is he satisfied with the time frame it takes to get payment? Does he have a good follow up system for payments? Is he filing electronically? Does he have any problem areas?

Does he have a lot of turnover of staff? Each time he loses his billing person, he has to find another and train her.

Check with each doctor you go to - your dentist, chiropractor, counselor, orthodontist, pediatrician, etc. Ask them if they know of any physicians who are having problems with their billing. Tell him you've started an electronic billing service and you are looking for clients. Ask if they have any suggestions.

2. *Spread the word.* Networking is absolutely the best way to find leads. Tell your friends, business associates, and acquaintances that you have started a new business and are looking for clients. Ask them if they know of any doctors' offices that have problems with the billing. Ask them if they will speak to their doctors about you. Offer them an incentive for any leads that turn into accounts. A gift certificate for a local restaurant is a great reward.

3. *Join networking groups,* business clubs, chamber of commerce, etc. You'll get to meet doctors, dentists, and therapists on a social level. They will be much more likely to be interested in what you do. Use the membership listings to find who is a potential client to target and then find a way to meet them.

4. *Mass marketing.* You can generate one letter in your computer and send it to all the physicians in your area. Make sure to send a well written letter and follow up a few days later with a phone call. Plan it to leave enough time to do all the follow up within a few days.

5. *Barter.* You may be seeing a provider who is willing to give you part or all of his insurance billing in trade for services. Even if you are not receiving cash, it is important to actually get the experience of doing some billing when you are getting your business started.

6. *Advertising.* It's a good idea to get your business name listed on Google. You may wish to purchase a little advertising space. You can also advertise your business in any local medical publications or the newspaper. And remember, your business is not limited to geographical location. Insurance claims can be submitted for a doctor in California even if the biller lives in New York. You may want to try advertising on the Internet.

7.   *Phone calls*. Some medical specialties such as social workers, chiropractors, etc. do not require employees. You can call their offices and leave an intriguing message on the answer phone telling them briefly about your service.

8. *Help wanted ads*. Follow the help wanted ads in the local newspaper. Watch for listings that are looking for medical billers. Be prepared to send a brochure and business cards. We even wrote up a resume for our company.

9. *New Practices*. Watch for new doctors starting their practice. They are the most likely to need help. Many new doctors are ill equipped to handle all the business obligations along with the patients and are glad to find help. You may have to do a little extra for them besides their insurance claims, but in the long run, it should be worth it. Check the newspapers for ads.

10. *Referrals*. Ask for referrals. Once you are working with a doctor and he is happy with your service, ask if he would be willing to refer you to any of his associates. As your business grows, you will find that your new business comes from referrals. Make sure you thank and reward the person who sent you the referral. They are very valuable to you. We also offer incentives for referrals.

Some of the girls who work in providers offices know others from different offices that might be interested. We've given gift certificates to a good local restaurant to people for giving referrals where we signed up the account.

11. *Brochures*. You may want to try walking into some of the potential doctors' offices with your brochures and see if you can talk to someone in charge. Be professional. Don't expect that you will be able to speak to the doctor, but if they are having a problem with their billing, they just might be willing to listen.

12. **_Website._** In this day and age a website is almost a requirement. This is your advertisement for your business so if you can't build a good professional looking site yourself you should consider hiring it done. Use other websites for ideas but make sure you don't copy any materials.

When you first start your marketing endeavor, it is a good idea to choose a medical field and target that one field. Specializing in one field makes good sense for many reasons. It is possible to become an expert in that specialty. This makes you valuable to other doctors in that field. There are a limited number of codes to learn. You only need to know the codes in that field, not the whole ICD10 and CPT books.

Eye doctors hang out with eye doctors, psychiatrists hang out with psychiatrists. The provider you are working for is more likely to refer you to another provider in the same field. Aggressively market this field. Don't sit and wait for a doctor to call you back because you left a message on his machine. Keep marketing. Find ways to meet professionals in your chosen field socially. You're much more likely to get their attention.

If you are not getting enough business from that field, pick one more and work that field also. But if you take on one chiropractor, one social worker, and one family doctor, you are going to have a lot more to learn.

If you need more ideas check out our books on marketing at www.medicalbillinglive.com.

What do you charge?

There are several ways to charge your clients. You can charge a monthly fee. When you don't have any experience yet, this can be difficult, because you will have no idea of how much work an account will be. The second way is a per claim fee. Many times, when sending the insurance claims is the only service you are providing, this can be the best way to charge. The average is from $3.00 to $8.00 per claim for an average provider. When you charge per claim, make sure you are clear on whether or not follow-up is expected and if secondary claims are included.

Most offices will hire a service because they also want the follow up taken care of as well as submitting the claims. Most people doing a full service find that a percentage of the income from insurance payments works best but unfortunately percentages are considered "fee splitting" and are against the law in several states.

Percentages will vary greatly. You should try to get an idea what providers in your area are paying. 5% to 8% seems to be the range. Usually when a percentage is charged the percentage is based upon what the provider actually collects as a result of the billing not the total amount billed out.

Many experienced billers will argue that percentage billing does not pay you for all the work you do. There is a lot of work done in the medical billing field that does not result in payment.

You may also want to consider a minimum monthly charge. We have a few accounts that are so small that they are not worth working with. Either they don't get a lot of insurance billing or they give us only one kind of insurance billing. A minimum fee helps to make this situation possible.

In some states charging a percentage is considered fee splitting and is illegal. Check with your attorney if you run into this problem. It is difficult to set a fee on work you have never done so give some major thought to how you are going to price your services.

We used to charge a percentage of what was collected, but found that we had to change our methods. New York is a fee splitting state and you can get your doctors in trouble charging that way. We now offer a flat monthly fee or a per claim fee based on the amount of claims they expect to send us.

In our contract with our providers, we state that we bill on the first of the month and payment to us is expected within 14 days. It is rare, but you may find that you have problems collecting from some of the providers. The services have already been provided deserve to be paid on time. You must act firmly with your clients about your pay. The longer you wait to take care of this problem, the worse it will get. We suggest a past due notice sent on the 15th of the month reminding them that payment is expected by the 14th.

For more information on how to charge your providers we have written an in-depth book on pricing your service called "Pricing Your Medical Billing Service".

Interviewing with a provider

Wow! You finally have an appointment with a provider. Remember, a provider is not always a doctor. Many providers that need medical billing done are not MD's. There are social workers, physical therapists, optometrists, etc.

One thing to remember when meeting with a provider is that they are a person just like you. Do not be intimidated by their title. They may be very good at what they do, and may have gone to school for a long time, but they need someone who knows about billing to take care of their receivables, and that someone can be you.

What to wear: Dress business like. First impressions are very important. This meeting is most likely what the provider will use to make his decision as to whether or not to hire you. You want to be neat and professional. You want your appearance to show him that you run a tight ship. Arrive a few minutes early, but not too early. Your time is valuable too.

What to take: We like to be totally prepared when we go on an interview. We usually take a contract with us filled out with the providers name and address and a form for all the information that is required to begin working for a provider.

There is quite a bit of information that is needed and you want to remember as much as possible. Our intention is to sign him up and we like to be prepared.

Also, in our folder we will have any paperwork we would need to file to get started. This may include a form to get permission to send the providers Medicare electronically and any forms from private insurances or the clearinghouse might require. A few business cards and a brochure will round it out. If you have any letters of referral from some of your existing clients, you may wish to bring copies of them.

Be confident: You will be providing a very good service, one that the provider needs. If he is already doing his billing in the office, you need to show him that you can do it more effectively and efficiently.

You are going to cut down on processing time, rejections, and claims that are "lost in the mail". You are also going to be able to follow up on claims faster because this is your only job. You don't have any patients to take care of, just the provider's billing. The more confident you look, the better your chances of getting hired.

This position is too important to not have someone who knows what they are doing - a professional. If it is a new provider, you can convince him that he is getting someone with experience. This will save him from having to hire someone and train them to do something that he knows nothing or little about. You can help him to get his practice going quicker.

Try to let the provider do most of the talking. Listen to what his or her needs are. Ask questions. Are they having any problems in particular? How would your service most benefit him?

It is easier to sell yourself when you know what their needs are. For example, if there is a high turnover rate, then you can emphasize that you are a reliable service that he can count on to be around. He won't have to bother interviewing any more people, and training them and hoping that they know what they are doing. Convince them that the receivables are too important to take a chance on.

Confidentiality is a major issue with many providers, especially with the HIPAA laws. The provider needs to be assured that his patient's information will not go beyond you and their records are kept in a secure area.

You must be very careful to not talk to anyone about any of your clients or their patients. And if you have anyone helping you, a confidentiality agreement must be signed.

If they decide to go ahead and sign your contract, complete the necessary paperwork, thank him or her for the decision, advise him or her on how long it will take to get the necessary paperwork to go through and determine when and how you will receive the first claims.

Contracts

One of the first questions most people have when they start a medical billing business is what do they use for a contract. Many people ask us for a copy of our contract so they can get an idea of what they want to say. We used to use a very simple one-page contract that really didn't say much. As we got more experience, we saw more things that we wanted included in our contract.

Remember that your contract is protecting you. When first starting out, you may not be sure of what you want to be protected from. As you grow, you see more things that should be covered in your contract.

One of the most important things your contract will cover is how you will be paid for your services. Many billing services charge a percentage of the money collected. Before you charge a percentage, make sure your state does not have "fee splitting" laws which prohibit a provider from sharing any percentage of his income with anyone outside of a partner. The states we are aware of that have fee splitting laws are NY, Fl, and NC but there are more.

Other methods of charging are a per claim fee, a flat fee, or a certain dollar per hour amount. However you have made arrangements to get paid it should be clearly spelled out in your contract.

The contract does not have to be a 20-page fine print legal document. It just has to state the important points regarding the relationship between you and the provider.

Whether you are taking over the billing from another service or the office has been doing it in-house, spell out the dates of service you will be responsible for. If a collection agency is used by the provider, your contract should specify if you will be reimbursed for any collections. Are you expected to clean up old billing that has not yet been paid? If you accept this type of work, how are you paid on that work? It is definitely more work than clean current billing so most billers charge more.

One of the most important items to cover in the contract is how your services will be terminated. How much notice must be given? You will want to specify a certain timeframe to allow for the change and to make sure you are paid for the work done.

The information you have received from the provider is the property of the doctor and is often expected to be returned to the doctor. This should be written into the contract. You might want to specify a timeframe for this also.

We highly recommend to not copy someone else's contract. You need to think your situation through and write down everything you can think of that could go wrong and cover it in your contract. Get your ideas together and take them to an attorney to write your contract.

In our book "Write a Kick Butt Contract For Your Medical Billing Service" we cover in depth all the things to consider when writing your contract. Some of the things we cover in this book are:

- Services you will provide
- How much will you charge
- Set up fee
- Minimum monthly charge
- Terms of the contract
- Confidentiality
- Effective date and identifying parties
- How and when the provider will pay you
- What are the provider's responsibilities?
- How HIPAA affects your contract
- Length of contract
- Termination
- Early termination
- Compliance plan
- How to find an attorney without costing you a lot

Working with your first doctor

So, you have your first account. The provider has decided to use your service. There is quite a bit of information that needs to be exchanged between the provider's office and your office.

You can build a form to take with you to fill in with the provider's name, title, address, phone number, fax number, specialty, any other office locations, tax id number, NPI #, Medicare number, Medicaid number, Workers' Comp number, office hours, which insurance companies they participates with, who you will be working with and the best time to reach them. Any numbers issued by private insurance companies, referred to as legacy numbers are generally not required since the use of NPI numbers.

You will also need a list of the CPT codes the doctor bills out with the charges they bill. Some providers use superbills which will contain all the CPT codes. If the office is not using a superbill or is a new provider without a system in place, you may be able to design a simple superbill for the office.

Establish a good relationship with the person you will work with in the office whether it is the provider, the spouse, receptionist, nurse, or office manager. Compliment them whenever possible. Tell the provider what a great job this person is doing - if they are.

This person could make you or break you. Occasionally you'll find it very difficult to work with someone. Try to stick it through for a while. Sometimes you can iron out the problems. Many times, these employees don't last long.

Most likely you will have some paperwork that the provider will have to sign including your contract with the provider. Also, Medicare requires the doctor's signature in order to bill electronically on his behalf. Our local Excellus BCBS requires the doctor to sign electronic contracts before claims can be submitted.

It is best to have all this paperwork completed as much as possible before asking the provider to sign. You don't want to be trying to figure out the forms in front of him. It will make it look like you don't know what you're doing.

Going to work
Starting a New Account

The contract is signed, the necessary numbers from the provider have been obtained, and your paperwork has been sent to the clearinghouse. The first thing that to do now is to find out when they want to start. Hopefully it will be immediately, but some may want to wait until the beginning of the month, or the quarter, or some other circumstance.

Assuming it is immediately, there is billing to do now. You will need to set up your software for the new provider. Consult your software manual for this information.

Start by adding a practice. Enter all of the provider's information into the software so that it will print out on the claims. This includes name and address, phone and fax numbers, tax id number, and NPI numbers.

Once this is done you may want to add the appropriate ICD10 and CPT codes for this specialty or your software may have the codes preloaded or the capability to import the codes.

You will also need to set up an electronic or paper filing system for the new account. You will need to develop a system. We set up a file for each provider with 3 folders in it. One for a copy of the contract and insurance forms, one for the patient's information forms and billing, and one for the EOBs.

Occasionally there is a need to go back to these files to retrieve something. What I recommend is always putting new papers in the back of the folder. That way you can try to retrieve things by date.

Develop a system for each provider on getting the necessary patient and claims information to your office. This can be done many ways, depending on the number of claims, location of offices, specialty, and provider's wishes.

Some providers expect billing to be done daily, some feel monthly is often enough. Most of our accounts are sent weekly with some of our larger accounts being bi-weekly or daily.

We receive claims information by mail, secure fax, secure email, pickup and drop-off. Each office can have a different method. Some of our providers are out of state and usually send us information by mail or fax or we download it from their computers.

We physically pick up information from our local offices once or twice a week. This works for us now, but we may find it easier to work with a courier in the future. A few offices fax, mail or email us the information weekly.

The important thing to remember here is to make it easy for your provider and your office. If they fax weekly and you don't receive a fax this week, make sure to call to find out why.

If you can't pick up on a scheduled day, call and let your provider know and make other arrangements. We pick up in one area on Mondays. Holidays such as Memorial Day and Labor Day always fall on Monday so we let them know we will see them on Tuesday.

We receive the information in many different forms. Some offices that are already using medical billing software find it easiest for them to just print CMS 1500 forms from their computers (on plain white paper to save costs) and send them to us. Other providers use a super bill. We have designed some of these super bills for them.

To a beginner, if a provider sends us a completed CMS form, it sometimes sounds like the provider's office has done all the work already. Nothing can be farther from the truth. Claims must be tracked and checked for proper payment. Just printing a CMS form and mailing it out is only a small part of what is required.

We enter the information from their forms into our computer and either send them electronically or print CMS 1500 forms to send on paper. If a provider is using a superbill, it is necessary to also submit a patient information form to us containing patient demographics and insurance information unless the superbill contains that information.

Superbills can range from very simple to very detailed depending on the providers specialty. Superbills must contain patient name, date of service, services provided (CPT4 codes), and diagnosis (ICD10 or ICD10 codes).

If the CMS forms are sent to us, it is not necessary to use a patient demographic form or a superbill as the CMS 1500 contains all the pertinent information. Once a patient is entered into our computer, we do not require the patient information sheet again. If the provider sees the patient on an ongoing basis, he will need to send only the claim information after the first time.

It is important to submit the insurance claims within 24 - 48 hours from when you receive the information from your client so the provider is paid as soon as possible.

Some providers will expect you to do their patient billing as well as insurance billing. This needs to be addressed when you and your client agree on your services. If they want you to do the patient billing, there are a few things you will need to consider. Your billing software should give you a few options of patient statements.

Decide with your provider how often you will be sending out these statements and exactly what information he or she wants printed on the statement. Determine how long to let an account go before it is necessary to send it to a collection agency. You may want to strike up a strategic alliance with a collection agency, as they sometimes have the opportunity to refer your services to a provider.

We use a three-statement patient billing policy. The first bill goes out with a detail of the charges and an explanation of what their portion is. You can purchase stickers with a variety of explanations, or you can make them up yourself with an inexpensive label program. Or you can print messages directly on your statements.

Here are some examples of our most commonly used notes or stickers:

"Your insurance has paid its portion of these charges.
 The balance is your responsibility."

"These charges have been applied to your deductible."

"Your insurance states your coverage has been terminated."

If there is no response to the first bill, we send out a second bill 30 days later. That bill we print in a balance forward format and add a note that says "2ND notice. We have not heard from you regarding your past due account."

If there is no response to the second bill, we send out a third and final bill 30 days after the second. That statement is also in the balance forward format and has a big orange sticker that says "Final Notice If payment is not received within 10 days, your account will be forwarded to collections"

This three-statement policy is what we recommend to our providers, but ultimately it is up to them how they want their patient billing handled. Make sure you discuss this with them prior to doing any patient billing.

Another little trick we learned with patient billing is that patients tend to pay quicker if you include a return envelope in with the statement. Many providers and services don't do this because they feel the envelopes cost too much. For the few pennies it costs for an envelope, the improved cash flow is well worth the expense.

We have a few very small accounts that we do patient billing. It isn't worth ordering 1000 return envelopes with their name and address so we simply make labels for these providers and apply them to small envelopes and insert them in the statements.

When we were a smaller company, we would take the patients statement and fold it so that the address shows through a window envelope with our return address preprinted. We then place the statement and the return envelope in the window envelope and mail it out. We now find it much more beneficial to use a company to send patient billing.

Pick a certain day of the month and designate it as your patient billing day. Pick a day that is not a busy time. For example, if you do your billing to your providers on the first of the month, you probably don't have time to do your patient billing then.

If you do your pickups on Monday, that probably wouldn't be good either. Consider making it the third Thursday every month. Having good systems in place when you first start out will help you to run smooth as you grow.

Aging Reports

Many people think that medical billing services just submit insurance claims for providers. They do that, but there is so much more. After the claims have been submitted, claims must be tracked to make sure they are paid on time. If a claim is not paid in 30 days (longer for workers' compensation) the insurance company needs to be contacted to see why it has not been paid. Some claim statuses can be checked online at the clearinghouse level or on the insurance carrier's websites. Others will require phone calls to the insurance carrier.

Rejection reports from the insurance carriers must be taken care of in the clearinghouse. When claims are submitted electronically, reports are received stating whether the claims were received, rejected or accepted and on some claims-specific rejection reasons.

It is important to understand all of the reports and how to read them so that any rejected claims can be handled. If it comes back rejected it is as if the insurance carrier never received the claim.

Another responsibility is reading the explanation of benefit statements (EOBs) and performing any necessary action. The EOB is the statement that accompanies payment or denial of payment from the insurance carrier. If it is processed correctly, the information is entered, however if it processed incorrectly, take further action must be taken.

Insurance companies do sometimes make mistakes in processing claims. When an error is found, a call must be made to straighten this out. A claim may be denied due to a coding error. If an outdated CPT code has been used, or an incorrect ICD10 code, the corrected claim must be submitted. The claim must be appealed. Another common denial is due to a request for additional information. This information must be obtained and forwarded on.

Sometimes a written appeal is necessary. If a claim has been denied for late submission, a brief explanation as to why the claim was not submitted on time must be sent to the insurance carrier with the denial and proof of the original submission.

On occasion a claim is denied because the insurance has been canceled. In this case, the provider must be notified immediately; or if you bill the patients, send the patient a statement advising them their insurance has denied their claim. It is your job to effectively read the EOB and act upon it to get the proper payment of each insurance claim for your client.

You can make yourself invaluable to your providers by your follow-up procedures. Set good procedures for follow-up right from the start and stick to them. Many providers don't have anyone in the office that really understands an EOB.

If you are unfamiliar with them, you should try to look at a couple to practice. If you have health insurance, you probably receive EOBs for your own family, but may never have paid much attention to them. Maybe your elderly parents get EOBs from their insurance. Try to look at as many as you can as EOBs vary greatly from one insurance to another.

Most insurance companies send statements to the insured even if the payment goes to the provider. Get a few out and study them. The more you read, the better you become. It is amazing that so many of the provider's staff do not know how to read these when they are so important. When you are trying to sell yourself to a provider, this can be one of your strong points.

Reports

The practice management software should be capable of generating several different reports. You will need to consult your software manual to see what reports are available to you. Some of the common ones are:

Insurance aging report - This report should list any outstanding insurance claims. Good software will sort the information in any way you wish. The aging report can be chosen by 30, 60, or 90 days and include or exclude certain data.

Patient aging report - This report will list any This report is run when sending the patient billing.

Day sheet - This report will list all activities done on an account for whatever specified time frame. We use this report to bill our providers for our services when charging a percentage. We print it out on the first of the month and use the totals at the bottom to show amounts collected that month.

There are several others that you may find quite helpful. Your providers may wish to receive some of these reports once or twice a month. This is an area you can use to make yourself invaluable to your provider. One thing we find in many offices is that even if they are using medical billing software, they do not know how to generate reports.

There is so much information that can be provided by reports. A monthly analysis or a yearly analysis can be run to let a provider know if they are on track. Or if not, where are they off?

Many providers are into the numbers and if you can provide them with the numbers, that makes them happy and it makes you look good. Familiarize yourself with your software's report capabilities.

HIPAA

HIPAA is the acronym for the Health Insurance Portability and Accountability Act of 1996. The Health Insurance Portability and Accountability Act of 1996 (HIPAA) mandated regulations that govern privacy, security, and electronic transactions standards for health care information.

These regulations have required major changes in how health care organizations handle all facets of information management, including reimbursement, coding, security, and patient records.

HIPAA calls for:

> 1. Standardization of electronic patient health, administrative and financial data

> 2. Unique health identifiers for individuals, employers, health plans and health care providers

> 3. Security standards protecting the confidentiality and integrity of "individually identifiable health information," past, present or future.

As a billing service, HIPAA did not impact us as much as the providers themselves, but it is important that you are HIPAA compliant as well.

If you are just setting your business up, these things are probably already taken care of, but you should ask anyway, just to make sure. Any records that you have need to be either in a locked filing cabinet, or unable to be accessed by any outsiders. Computers should be password protected.

You and any employees will need to understand the importance of confidentiality. Also, you should be able to advise your providers if they are breaking any HIPAA rules.

As a medical billing service, you also need to name a HIPAA Compliance Officer. If you are a one-man band then obviously the HIPAA Compliance Officer will be you. It is still important that you formally name yourself as the Compliance Officer anyway. Any complaints or HIPAA violations are filed through the Compliance Officer.

The following are some good informational websites regarding HIPAA:

http://www.hipaa-iq.com
http://www.hcfa.gov/hipaa/hipaahm.htm
http://www.hipaadvisory.com/

NPI Numbers

NPI or National Provider Numbers were implemented on May 23, 2007. Each provider must have an NPI number to identify themselves. Previous to the NPI number system, each insurance company would identify a provider with an individual legacy number.

In an effort to simplify healthcare administration each healthcare provider must obtain a free NPI number from the NPI enumerator to identify him/herself. Without this NPI identification number printed on insurance claim forms claims will be denied.

The original deadline for this requirement of the NPI numbers on insurance claims was May 23, 2007 but was extended to May 23, 2008 as many companies were not ready by the original deadline.

Any provider who is paid by insurance carriers for medical insurance claims or refers patients to specialists for treatment must obtain an NPI number. A tax id number is also required besides the NPI number on all insurance claims. One of the services we offer as a billing service is that we will obtain the NPI number for our providers.

There are two types of NPI numbers. Type I or individual NPI numbers and Type II NPI numbers are for providers who bill using a legal business name and EIN number.

Insurances

There are two general categories of health insurance, public and private. Public health insurances consists of Medicare, Medicaid, Champus (government insurance), and various others. Private health insurance consists primarily of commercial companies, including, Blue Cross Blue Shield plans, United Healthcare, AETNA, CIGNA and Health Maintenance Organizations (HMO's).

In many of both public and private insurances, a provider can be either participating or non-participating. This means that he can choose to accept a company's guidelines and fees for services or not. If he or she chooses to, they become a participating provider with that company. Some benefits of participating are: payment is sent directly to the provider (instead of the patient), being listed in the company directory, claims receive priority in processing over non-participating providers, higher fee schedules in some cases, and lower out of pocket expenses for patients with that insurance.

Some disadvantages of participating are: accepting the fee schedule and treatment being dictated. The disadvantage of not participating is patients may receive little or no reimbursement for services and may choose to go elsewhere.

Each carrier differs dramatically in their fee schedules, and in their requirements for participation, treatment authorization, and claims filing. Providers may choose to participate with some and not with others and may look to their biller for advice in making this decision. It helps to know the requirements and fee schedules of common insurance carriers.

Most carriers have a timely filing deadline. That means that there is a designated amount of time from the date of service in which you have to file the claim. The deadline varies greatly from company to company. Some have a deadline from as little as 30 days from the date of service and others can go up to 2 years. It is important to know the filing deadline for each carrier.

The patient can authorize payment to go directly to the provider by signing an assignment of benefits statement. If the provider participates with an insurance carrier, in most cases, the payment will automatically go to the provider, whether the patient signs a statement or not.

But some companies will only send the money to the provider if they have a signed statement on file. This statement can be as simple as a line on the bottom of the patient information form that states "I authorize payment for services to be sent directly to <fill in provider's name>." This assignment of benefits is indicated in box 13 on the CMS 1500 form.

It also important to have the patient sign a statement indicating that the provider has permission to release any medical information to the insurance carrier that is necessary to receive payment for the services provided.

For instance, if the insurance carrier requests medical records in order to determine if a service is going to be covered, the provider needs the patient's permission to send the records to the insurance carrier.

Again, this can just be a simple line along with the assignment of benefits statement that is something like "I authorize the release of any information to the insurance carrier regarding my treatment."

Many patients are required by the insurance carrier to pay a portion of their bill in the form of either a co-payment or co-insurance. If the patient has an HMO, they will have a designated co-payment that they are required to pay.

Some insurance plans require that the patient meet a deductible each year. This deductible must be satisfied by the patient before the insurance company will begin making payments on their claims. The patient is responsible for this amount and deductibles vary from plan to plan.

It is a good idea to familiarize yourself with the major insurance companies for your area. Most commercial insurance companies have provider representatives. Find out who your area provider rep is and make contact with them to introduce yourself.

Medicare, Medicaid and many commercial carriers publish monthly bulletins or newsletters for the providers containing updates and changes. It is important to keep up with this information.

A call can be made to the Medicare & Medicaid offices to get on the mailing list for these bulletins or ask one of your providers to save them for you when they are finished. Many of the bulletins or newsletters are available online.

It is a possible that a patient may be eligible for two separate insurance plans. One would be primary and should be billed first and the other would be secondary. Insurance companies determine which policy is primary through a method called COB, or coordination of benefits.

There are a couple of different methods to determine which insurance policy is primary. If a husband and a wife both work and both have family insurance policies, their own insurance will be primary and their spouse's insurance will be secondary.

When children are involved, one method used to determine who is primary is called the birthday rule. That is where the insurance plan of whichever person's month of birth is earlier would be primary. (If they are born in the same month they go on to the day of birth.)

Another method, called the gender rule, states that the male person's insurance plan is primary. Yet another would be if a person had two insurance plans themselves, one from a company that they are currently working for, and one that they are retired from, the insurance plan for the current employer would be primary.

If a person had an insurance plan and also Medicaid, Medicaid is always secondary to the other plan, no matter what company it is. When a patient has Medicare, Medicare is prime unless the patient or the patient's spouse is currently employed and has insurance coverage through that employer. The patient's coverage through the company of the employed person would be primary and Medicare would be secondary.

There is one exception to this rule. That is if the employed group insures less than 100 people, then Medicare would be prime even though either the patient, or the patient's spouse is employed. Medicare would have to contact the other insurance carrier to get the information straight.

There are some other methods of determining COB, but these are the most commonly used.

After receiving the EOB from the primary company, a claim must be printed on another CMS 1500 for the secondary company. Attach the primary company's EOB and mail it.

Medicare has a program called Medigap which automatically forwards claims information electronically to secondary carriers able to receive claims. If Medicare forwards the claim automatically, it will indicate that it was forwarded and to what insurance carrier right on the Medicare Explanation of Benefits Statement. Many insurance companies can now receive even secondary claims electronically.

Claims - Paper Vs. Electronic

There are many advantages to sending insurance claims electronically instead of on paper. Electronic claims processing (ECP) saves time, labor, money and paper. Many insurance carriers including Medicare are now requiring electronic submissions and don't allow paper claims without a special waiver.

There is no need to print up a CMS 1500, just type the information into the practice management program in the computer. The claim can actually be received by the insurance company within 24 hours.

ECP cuts down on much overhead for insurance companies and a few companies are trying to mandate ECP and are offering many incentives.

Some providers are still looking into ways to send their claims electronically. In order to send claims electronically from their offices, they must have a fairly up-to-date computer, high speed modem, appropriate software, clearinghouse connection and an employee who knows how to operate all this. You can show them that your service saves them the work of updating their office and having an employee who is capable of electronic billing.

A paper claim must go through many steps before it reaches the person who is responsible for paying the claim. The claim is first sorted and routed, microfilmed and batched. They are then keyed into a computer, examined by an auditor, and accepted or rejected.

Electronic claims can be processed much quicker and with fewer steps. Payment is much quicker when claims are submitted electronically.

Summary

We hope we have been helpful in giving a full picture of what it takes to start and run a medical billing business. The experience of others can be very beneficial to many going through the same issues and it is our desire to help those questioning whether or not a medical billing business is something that they could do successfully. There is no question in our minds that it is possible. We did it and we have met, watched, and helped many others succeed.

Starting a medical billing service is definitely not a get rich quick scheme. It is like any other business, lots of hard work. It takes a certain kind of person to overcome the obstacles and work through the issues. You need determination and a willingness to do what it takes. For most beginners the most difficult part of starting a medical billing business is finding clients. So, one of the most important parts to success is a willingness to do what it takes to find clients.

Marketing is vital to growing a medical billing service. The largest reason for failure is a lack of marketing. A person considering this field must learn to market their services. There are many different marketing methods and we offer three books on marketing to help with this challenge.

A medical billing service is a very flexible business that can serve as a supplemental income for a person who just wants a little extra income or it can be a business with many employees. This business can become whatever you want it to.

If you have decided that this is the business for you, we have written several other books that may be of help to you. We are also offering an online course in medical billing to give you the opportunity to learn exactly what a medical biller needs to know to either hold a medical billing position or to build a business. We wish you the best of success in your undertaking.

Terminology

Allowable Amount -   the maximum amount that the insurance carrier will consider reimbursing for a covered service or procedure.

Authorizations - prior approval of payment by the insurance carrier to the provider for services to a patient

Beneficiary - a person eligible for benefits under a health insurance plan

Clearinghouse - A company which will receive electronic insurance claims, sort and reroute them to the proper carriers

Co-insurance - Portion of the insurance bill remaining after the carrier has made payment on a claim that is the patient's responsibility

Coordination of Benefits - Method of determining which insurance carrier is primary for a patient when more than one insurance is involved

Co-pay - Amount that patient is required to pay for each visit or service performed by a provider

CPT Codes - Physicians' Current Procedural Terminology is a listing of descriptive terms and identifying codes for reporting medical services and procedures

Crossover - Automatic forwarding of claim information from Medicare to a patient's secondary insurance carrier

Deductible - a specified amount of money that the insured must pay before an insurance carrier will make payments on any claims

Electronic claims processing - The process of submitting insurance claims electronically

Explanation of benefits (EOB)- Statement which accompanies payment or denial of payment from an insurance company

ICD10 Codes - International classification of diseases codes for purposes of diagnosis

ERA - Electronic Remittance Notice, an electronic version of the EOB or Explanation of Benefits Statement. ERA's are received as an electronic file either thru a clearinghouse or directly from the insurance carrier.

Fee Schedule - a complete list of fees that a medical provider charges for each service they provide

Insurance Carrier - Insurance Company

Intake Form - a form used to collect information from a patient including demographics and insurance information needed for the purpose of billing and claims submission

Medigap - Medicare program that automatically electronically transfers claims information to secondary carriers

Modifiers - A two digit extension to a CPT code that further explains procedure or service performed

No fault - Insurance claims resulting from an automobile accident

Patient Responsibility - the amount of money that the patient is liable for after the insurance carrier has processed their claim

Pre-Authorization -   indication from the insurance carrier that certain medical services will be covered for a patient (Please note that Pre-authorization is not a guarantee that the claim will be paid.)

Provider - an individual or an institution that provides preventive, curative, promotional, or rehabilitative health care services in a systematic way to individuals, families or communities

Referrals - Notification from a patient's primary care physician for permission to go to a specialist (This is not always an authorization or a guarantee of payment)

Reimbursement - compensation or repayment for healthcare services rendered

Superbill - A form used in a provider's office to document the patient's visit

Treatment notes (Soap notes) - Patient's progress notes

Usual and Customary - the allowance for each medical service determined by an insurance carrier based on claim data collected by the insurance carrier for the same medical service based on a provider's geographical region

Workers Comp - Insurance claims resulting directly from a work-related illness or injury

Abbreviations

Auth/Ref - Authorization or referral

BC/BS - Blue Cross Blue Shield

BTW – Back to work

CAP - Claims Assistant Professional

CHAMPUS - Civilian health and medical program of the uniformed services

CMS – Centers for Medicare and Medicaid Services

COB - Coordination of Benefits

CPT codes – procedural medical code

Ded - Deductible

DOB - Date of Birth

DOS - Date of Service

DTW - Deep tissue work

Dx - Diagnosis codes

ECP - Electronic claims processing

EOB - Explanation of benefits

EOMB - Explanation of Medicare Benefits

ER - Emergency room

HCFA – Health Care Financing Administration

HCPCS – HCFA common procedure coding system

HIPAA – Health Insurance Portability and Accountability Act of 1996

HMO – Health Maintenance Organization

H & P – History & Physical

Lt – Left

MH – Mental Health

NF – No Fault

Non-par – Non=participating provider

OTR – Outpatient treatment report

PAR – Participating provider

PCP – Primary care physician

PI – Personal injury

POS – Place of service

PPO – Preferred provider organization

Pt – Patient

PT – Physical therapist

RNC – Reasonable, Necessary & Customary

ROM – Range of motion

Rt – Right

RTW – Return to work

Rx – Prescription for treatment

SOAP –

SOF – Signature on file

TX – therapy

UPIN – Unique Physician Identification Number

WC – Workers Compensation

2X – 2 Times

2X/wk – 2 times per week

Other books available by Alice Scott and Michele Redmond

"Basics of Medical Billing" - Instantly Improve the efficiency and cash flow of your office using this guide! It's a must read for everyone from the receptionist to the doctor in any medical office!

"12 Marketing Strategies to Grow Your Medical Billing Business" – written in 2002 and revised several times. If you've started your medical billing service and need to find more clients, you **need** this book.

"Take Your Medical Billing Business To The Next Level" – Are you ready to expand your medical billing business? Are you ready to take on more business or hire an employee? Here are the secrets we've learned in the last 17 years from starting our own medical billing business to currently billing for over fifty providers.

"Secrets to Signing Up Your First Doctor" – Learn the secrets to finding and signing up your first accounts.

"How to Complete a UB04 Form Completely and Correctly" – Complete instructions on completing a UB04 form correctly so your claims will be paid on the first submission.

"How To Complete a CMS 1500 Completely and Correctly - Line By Line, Box By Box" Complete instructions on completing a CMS 1500 form correctly in easy to understand language.

"Introduction to Chiropractic Billing" – How to make sure your claims are paid properly and you are reimbursed completely for your chiropractic services.

"Introduction to Mental Health Billing" – How to make sure your claims are paid properly and you are reimbursed completely for your mental health services. Whether you are a social worker, a psychologist, a psychiatrist or a psychoanalyst, this book can teach you exactly how to bill out and get paid for your services.

"Write a Kick Butt Contract for Your Medical Billing Service"– East to follow instructions that walk you step by step through the process of writing a contract for your medical billing service, even if you have no idea where to start! We show you what you need to consider when writing a contract, scenarios of situations that can arise as well as sample wording to use <u>while saving you a ton of money in lawyer's fees!</u>

"Pricing Your Medical Billing Service" - Guide to the commonly used methods of charging for your services with the pros and cons. Make sure you are not breaking the law with one commonly used method. This book breaks down all the services you may wish to charge for.

"Denials, Appeals & Adjustments" – A step by step guide to handling denied medical insurance claims, when and how to appeal a denied claim and how and when to make adjustments to processed insurance claims.

"Advanced Medical Billing Marketing for the New Economy" – This book examines effective marketing ideas for this tough economy and gives the reader a toolbox of methods to reach their market.

"Introduction to Physical Therapy, Occupational Therapy and Speech Therapy Billing" - Whether you are a therapy office looking to have a better understanding of the billing process, an established billing service looking to expand your billing specialties or a new biller trying to get started in the field of therapy, this book will give you an introduction to the "ins and outs" of therapy billing.

Made in the USA
Monee, IL
10 December 2024

72916277R00044